UOM, Inc Tree House Ministry Products are available at special quality for bulk purchases for the sale and promotional premium fundraisers and educational needs.

For more details write: 3615 Victory Blvd, Ste 105 Portsmouth, Virginia 23701 stacy.coward@yahoo.com (757)581-3897

Copyright 2022 by UOM, Inc Tree House Ministry Products .This edition published in 2022

Compiled and edited by Tree House Ministry

Design by UOM, Inc Tree House Ministry Products: ISBN 978-1-4583-4735-0
Imprint: Lulu.com

The Art of Loving Yourself

GRATITUDE PLANNER

A Practical Tool for Planning Your Life

Dr. Stacy D. Coward ThD, LPC, RN

UOM, Inc

Tree House Ministries

DEDICATED

To those who are trying to organized their lives

to create the greatest version of themselves

HOW TO USE THIS PLANNER

Use this planner to consider your life from the perspective of gratitude. We all are going through something at one time or another. The goal is to lean in on the hard times and face the rougher times with an attitude of gratitude. Learning to be thankful in all things, ways, days, and phases help to make the journey lighter. THANK YOU is a gift that goes a long way both in the spiritual and natural realms.

This planner will help keep you a place of Gratitude and Thanksgiving

THROUGHOUT THE PLANNER YOU WILL HAVE AN OPPORTUNITY TO

ACTIVATE YOUR VOICE POWER BY SAYING THANK YOU IT WILL BE

PROMPTED BY THE WORDS

Now Say.....

THANK YOU

Author's Note

Many people go through many things during this journey but very few people understand the power in a "THANK YOU" that helps to make the journey easier.

INTRODUCTION

Live in an Attitude of Gratitude

Our family dog Rosebud is such a wonderful example of living for an Attitude of Gratitude. I call her our guardian angels assigned to us throughout eternity. Sometimes, when I talk to her I tell her I know she is a great white lion that has always been around to cover and protect us. She loves us so much. She is always so thankful for everything. She shows us so must thanks by jumping up and down, smiling, barking in a high pitched voice, hopping around like a rabbit and even dancing on two feet when she sees us. She does all of this to say I am so glad to see you. She makes us feel as though we are the most important people in the world and she is so grateful to be with us. She always greets us at the door. If we forget to say goodbye she stands in the door screen watching us drive away. She sleeps right next to the bed while always making sure we are guarded and protection from any strange noise or movement outside.

Rosebud is the epitome of what being thankful for whom you have been assigned to looks like. She is loyal, unfailing, consistent and always grateful for even the slightest attention. Rosebud reminds me how to show that I am grateful and how to authentically love. Lord I THANK YOU for my Rose buddy!

Teach us to be more grateful and show more unconditional love for each other.

Key Terms

THANK YOU is a polite expression when used acknowledging a gift, service, or complement. It facilitates a calm, reasoned and respectful discussion. Even when there is a difference on viewpoints it creates civility when there are disagreements.

A realm is something that is governed by a set of rules or a ruler that makes the rules.

FOREWORD

I know that it can be a challenge being thankful when things are hard. Over the years, I have faced many challenges but one of the greatest gifts that I have learned to use and operate from is praise. When I open up my mouth to say THANK YOU it activates places that I cannot reach with my hands, money, strategies, education, relationships, and so many other resources that we attempt to employ in times of need or adversity. I have learned that the THANK YOU is a big part of what I need to move past many hard places in life. The reason why I can sit still in a place of praise when I say THANK YOU is because I understand that everything that I am or hope to be is in the hands of the Lord. He is the good Shepherd. He is the way maker. He is my provider.

As I teach you to use your gift of praise by using the words THANK YOU, you will become more empowered to embrace your changes, obstacles and new way of thinking. There are no mistakes everything that you have faced in life will all be used for your good. You are not alone and although it may not seem like it sometimes things are working out for your good! Now Say , THANK YOU !"

Using the words THANK YOU has its greatest impact when it comes from a place of a surrendered heart. Knowing that you belong to something much bigger than yourself and everything that concerns you concerns that Higher Power you are able to rest and connect your heart THANK YOU to your head THANK YOU. It is more than just saying the words thank you. It is your capacity to understand and believe that the THANK YOU is actually activating something in other realms. I believe I have the power to praise my way to wherever I'm trying to go. THANK YOU is the fuel for the journey.

SCRIPTURE REFERENCE

Psalm 23 King James Version (KJV)

The Lord is my shepherd; I shall not want. He maketh me to lie down in green pastures: he leadeth me beside the still waters. He restoreth my soul: he leadeth me in the paths of righteousness for his name's sake. Yea, though I walk through the valley of the shadow of death, I will fear no evil: for thou art with me; thy rod and thy staff they comfort me. Thou prepares a table before me in the presence of mine enemies: thou anointest my head with oil; my cup runneth over. Surely goodness and mercy shall follow me all the days of my life: and I will dwell in the house of the Lord forever.

Now let us get started on this season by activating your promises through the use of the two simple but powerful words –

THANK YOU

The difference between those people who continue to grow, thrive and maintain verses everyone else is their Consistent Attitude of Gratitude

IMPORTANT DAYS TO REMEMBER THIS YEAR

Monday	Tuesday	Wednesday	Thursday	Friday	Saturday	Sunday

IMPORTANT DAYS TO REMEMBER THIS YEAR

Monday	Tuesday	Wednesday	Thursday	Friday	Saturday	Sunday

_____

_____

_____

_____

_____

_____

IMPORTANT DAYS TO REMEMBER THIS YEAR

Monday	Tuesday	Wednesday	Thursday	Friday	Saturday	Sunday

_____

_____

_____

_____

_____

Monday	Tuesday	Wednesday	Thursday	Friday	Saturday	Sunday

IMPORTANT DAYS TO REMEMBER THIS YEAR

Your ability to readjust your attitude throughout the day, moment, and seasons of your life will be your saving grace.

*	TO DO LIST FOR THE WEEK	FOLLOW UP

Mindfulness Technique for using Thank YOU:

Your mind, body and soul interface all the time

Spend your early waking hours in a **Mental Posture** of Thanksgiving (**MIND**) before you do anything else. Your heart (**BODY**) will take on the posture of humility and your emotions (**SOUL**) will create a space for Angels to operate in the will of God on your behalf as you focus on gratitude

IMPORTANT DAYS TO REMEMBER THIS WEEK

Monday	Tuesday	Wednesday	Thursday	Friday	Saturday	Sunday

SELF TALK

Create a POSITIVE NARRATIVE over your life

Life and Death are in the power of your tongue. You can speak LIFE over your situation just by saying

THANK YOU

Have you ever consider that perhaps some of the things that you wanted in life you were not ready to receive all the responsibilities that came along with the blessing?

When we do not understand what is happening a **THANK YOU** is always an appropriate response!

Activation power of a **THANK YOU**

We should continually be in a place of thanksgiving. Even when we do not understand, a **THANK YOU** goes a long way in the spirit realm. **THANK YOU** will assist you in manifesting the necessary tools, knowledge, maturity and experiences to gain what you need to be prepared to receive the gifts in the natural realm.

When in doubt break out into a praise! It will carry you a long, long way!

Monday	Tuesday	Wednesday	Thursday	Friday	Saturday	Sunday

Write down as many reasons to be grateful at this very present moment

Learning how to say **THANK YOU** is one of the most powerful tools you can establish as a foundational pillar.

Monday	Tuesday	Wednesday	Thursday	Friday	Saturday	Sunday

When you speak the words **THANK YOU** it covers many areas of your life.

Monday	Tuesday	Wednesday	Thursday	Friday	Saturday	Sunday

We should remain in a spirit or attitude of gratitude because our very cells respond to the position of thankfulness.

Monday	Tuesday	Wednesday	Thursday	Friday	Saturday	Sunday

THANK YOU is the universal language that transcends words. It sets up a spiritual connection between you, people, items, experiences, hopes, dreams, visions and anything else you can think of that you are grateful towards.

Monday	Tuesday	Wednesday	Thursday	Friday	Saturday	Sunday

Some important keys to remember it is one thing to say it but it is a whole another power to believe it. I believe wholeheartedly that my words have significant power and as I speak the words **THANK YOU** it means that I believe God to move on my behalf as the good Shepherd.

Key Number One

My head talk and my heart talk have to match

Key Number Two

The Lord is my shepherd I shall not want **for anything**

Key Number Three

I am able to partner with God's angels to orchestrate the life that God has planned for me

Key Number Four

The Angels that are assigned to my life cannot move on some things on my behalf until I activate them through my praise

Use the GRATITUDE method of meditation for the next 30 days to create a life time habit.

Write down as many reasons to be grateful at this very present moment

THANK YOU

Spirit Realm

THANK YOU is the button that is pushed to start the angels moving on your behalf

JOT DOWN THINGS YOU NEED ANGELIC HELP TO ACCOMPLISH

Now Say.......

THANK YOU

THANK YOU voice prints the walls of your environment with praise so God will inhabit the areas that you dwell in.

Monday	Tuesday	Wednesday	Thursday	Friday	Saturday	Sunday

VOICE PRINT YOUR WALLS THROUGH A THANK YOU

WRITE DOWN WHAT YOU WILL SPEAK TO THE ATOMS OF YOUR WALLS

THEY ARE ALIVE AND STORE INFORMATION

THANK YOU establishes the provisions for the assignment of your hands

Monday	Tuesday	Wednesday	Thursday	Friday	Saturday	Sunday

THANK YOU is the voice command that tells the angels in heaven to start the process of healing.

Monday	Tuesday	Wednesday	Thursday	Friday	Saturday	Sunday

THANK YOU gives you protection

Monday	Tuesday	Wednesday	Thursday	Friday	Saturday	Sunday

THANK YOU causes the need for the day to be sent forth and find you.

Monday	Tuesday	Wednesday	Thursday	Friday	Saturday	Sunday

THANK YOU
Written Realm

THANK YOU creates the letters of gratitude that are needed to be written from the heavenly realms on your behalf.

Monday	Tuesday	Wednesday	Thursday	Friday	Saturday	Sunday

THANK YOU creates a formal business agreement that is

activated by your praise

Monday	Tuesday	Wednesday	Thursday	Friday	Saturday	Sunday

THANK YOU covers up old traditions and establishes a new way of doing things.

Monday	Tuesday	Wednesday	Thursday	Friday	Saturday	Sunday

THANK YOU causes a recognition of formality to be seen coming from you

Monday	Tuesday	Wednesday	Thursday	Friday	Saturday	Sunday

THANK YOU creates hand written letters from your perspective

Monday	Tuesday	Wednesday	Thursday	Friday	Saturday	Sunday

THANK YOU creates a connection between your feelings, behaviors and your emotions

Monday	Tuesday	Wednesday	Thursday	Friday	Saturday	Sunday

THANK YOU can be sent to your significant other from the spiritual domain to another domain.

Monday	Tuesday	Wednesday	Thursday	Friday	Saturday	Sunday

THANK YOU puts wings on the need for the day so it can hurry up and get to you

Monday	Tuesday	Wednesday	Thursday	Friday	Saturday	Sunday

Now Say.......

THANK YOU

THANK YOU causes multiplication of whatever you lack.

Monday	Tuesday	Wednesday	Thursday	Friday	Saturday	Sunday

THANK YOU causes angels to whisper creative witty ideas in your ears as you sleep

Monday	Tuesday	Wednesday	Thursday	Friday	Saturday	Sunday

THANK YOU

Emotional Realm

THANK YOU realigns your mind and your mouth

Monday	Tuesday	Wednesday	Thursday	Friday	Saturday	Sunday

THANK YOU causes you to sends a signal to every part of your body that whatever the issue was it is taken care of.

Monday	Tuesday	Wednesday	Thursday	Friday	Saturday	Sunday

THANK YOU commands your mind not to wander off in doubt and remain subject to your mouth

Monday	Tuesday	Wednesday	Thursday	Friday	Saturday	Sunday

THANK YOU commands your body to function as though the provision is already there.

Monday	Tuesday	Wednesday	Thursday	Friday	Saturday	Sunday

THANK YOU
Universe Realm

THANK YOU sends a signal out into the universe stating, "I know that my needs have already been taken care of and I know help is on the way!"

Monday	Tuesday	Wednesday	Thursday	Friday	Saturday	Sunday

THANK YOU causes the universe to send forth the missing piece because you are operating as though you already have it.

Monday	Tuesday	Wednesday	Thursday	Friday	Saturday	Sunday

THANK YOU activates the universe to send the provision in your life

Monday	Tuesday	Wednesday	Thursday	Friday	Saturday	Sunday

THANK YOU ignites the universal laws to give you more of what you desire

Monday	Tuesday	Wednesday	Thursday	Friday	Saturday	Sunday

THANK YOU raises your vibrations in the universe to move whatever you need towards you

Monday	Tuesday	Wednesday	Thursday	Friday	Saturday	Sunday

THANK YOU is the wheel that makes your life continue to have momentum

Monday	Tuesday	Wednesday	Thursday	Friday	Saturday	Sunday

THANK YOU
Natural Realm

DID YOU KNOW: Your body is 70 percent water? Studies have shown that you can speak to molecules of water and cause them to appear differently. Dark for negative talk or crystallized for positive talk.

Monday	Tuesday	Wednesday	Thursday	Friday	Saturday	Sunday

Write down as many reasons to be grateful at this very present moment

_____

_____

_____

_____

_____

_____

_____

Now Say.......

THANK
YOU

THANK YOU shifts your molecules in your body to a crystallized state

Monday	Tuesday	Wednesday	Thursday	Friday	Saturday	Sunday

THANK YOU causes the ions in your cells to change from negative to positive

Monday	Tuesday	Wednesday	Thursday	Friday	Saturday	Sunday

THANK YOU causes positive people, places and things to happen to you

Monday	Tuesday	Wednesday	Thursday	Friday	Saturday	Sunday

THANK YOU makes your body function better

Monday	Tuesday	Wednesday	Thursday	Friday	Saturday	Sunday

THANK YOU
Faith Realm

THANK YOU is the water that is needed to make your faith grow

Monday	Tuesday	Wednesday	Thursday	Friday	Saturday	Sunday

THANK YOU means that you believe it is already done

Monday	Tuesday	Wednesday	Thursday	Friday	Saturday	Sunday

Now Say.......

THANK YOU

THANK YOU is said after someone gives you something

Monday	Tuesday	Wednesday	Thursday	Friday	Saturday	Sunday

THANK YOU is your way of using your mouth in faith

Monday	Tuesday	Wednesday	Thursday	Friday	Saturday	Sunday

THANK YOU aligns your thinking to know that whatever you need is already done. There is an expected ending. You are no longer hoping but knowing that you have been given what you ask the Lord for

Monday	Tuesday	Wednesday	Thursday	Friday	Saturday	Sunday

THANK YOU says I trust you Lord

Monday	Tuesday	Wednesday	Thursday	Friday	Saturday	Sunday

THANK YOU says we don't have to worry about this because it was taken care of

Monday	Tuesday	Wednesday	Thursday	Friday	Saturday	Sunday

THANK YOU says stop crying God has handled all of your needs

Monday	Tuesday	Wednesday	Thursday	Friday	Saturday	Sunday

THANK YOU

Future Realm

THANK YOU blesses your grandchildren

Monday	Tuesday	Wednesday	Thursday	Friday	Saturday	Sunday

THANK YOU blesses 3-4 generations after you

Monday	Tuesday	Wednesday	Thursday	Friday	Saturday	Sunday

THANK YOU activates the vision of your future

Monday	Tuesday	Wednesday	Thursday	Friday	Saturday	Sunday

THANK YOU establishes new foundation to hope in

Monday	Tuesday	Wednesday	Thursday	Friday	Saturday	Sunday

THANK YOU creates the seeds you have planted

Monday	Tuesday	Wednesday	Thursday	Friday	Saturday	Sunday

THANK YOU summons help from your future

Monday	Tuesday	Wednesday	Thursday	Friday	Saturday	Sunday

THANK YOU causes the path pointers to give you direction

Monday	Tuesday	Wednesday	Thursday	Friday	Saturday	Sunday

Write down as many reasons to be grateful at this very present moment

_____

_____

_____

_____

_____

_____

_____

THANK YOU
Hope Realm

THANK YOU increases your longevity

Monday	Tuesday	Wednesday	Thursday	Friday	Saturday	Sunday

THANK YOU lives past you

Monday	Tuesday	Wednesday	Thursday	Friday	Saturday	Sunday

THANK YOU is the signature of completion that says, "I am finished and I command this work to continue to stand long after I am gone!"

Monday	Tuesday	Wednesday	Thursday	Friday	Saturday	Sunday

THANK YOU says, "I have no more to say." It is done.

Monday	Tuesday	Wednesday	Thursday	Friday	Saturday	Sunday

THANK YOU calls your blessing to come upon those people you value creates the momentum for your legacy

Monday	Tuesday	Wednesday	Thursday	Friday	Saturday	Sunday

THANK YOU
Energy Realm

THANK YOU causes positive energy to be gathered into one space near you

Monday	Tuesday	Wednesday	Thursday	Friday	Saturday	Sunday

Write down as many reasons to be grateful at this very present moment

_____

_____

_____

_____

_____

_____

_____

Now Say.......

THANK YOU

THANK YOU releases positive energy from your body

Monday	Tuesday	Wednesday	Thursday	Friday	Saturday	Sunday

THANK YOU creates a magnetic force to surround you 3 meters around your body

Monday	Tuesday	Wednesday	Thursday	Friday	Saturday	Sunday

THANK YOU helps you to maintain the momentum to finish

Monday	Tuesday	Wednesday	Thursday	Friday	Saturday	Sunday

THANK YOU releases you from energy of the memories that captivate your mind

Monday	Tuesday	Wednesday	Thursday	Friday	Saturday	Sunday

THANK YOU releases you from the negative energy of the people around you

Gratitude Planner
A Practical Tool for Planning Your Life

Monday	Tuesday	Wednesday	Thursday	Friday	Saturday	Sunday

THANK YOU
Mind Realm

THANK YOU allows your mind to be free to think

Monday	Tuesday	Wednesday	Thursday	Friday	Saturday	Sunday

THANK YOU focuses your attention on gratitude for your life

Monday	Tuesday	Wednesday	Thursday	Friday	Saturday	Sunday

THANK YOU resets your thinking to an attitude of gratitude in the moment of crisis

Monday	Tuesday	Wednesday	Thursday	Friday	Saturday	Sunday

THANK YOU causes witty inventions to be released to your mind

Monday	Tuesday	Wednesday	Thursday	Friday	Saturday	Sunday

THANK YOU opens portals to your mind

Monday	Tuesday	Wednesday	Thursday	Friday	Saturday	Sunday

THANK YOU allows you to dream a new dream

Monday	Tuesday	Wednesday	Thursday	Friday	Saturday	Sunday

THANK YOU
Vision Realm

THANK YOU makes you envision your body in optimal working condition

Monday	Tuesday	Wednesday	Thursday	Friday	Saturday	Sunday

Now Say.......

THANK YOU

THANK YOU allows you to see the vision for your family

Monday	Tuesday	Wednesday	Thursday	Friday	Saturday	Sunday

THANK YOU allows you to see your hands grasping your future

Monday	Tuesday	Wednesday	Thursday	Friday	Saturday	Sunday

THANK YOU allows you to see your feet walking on the correct path

Monday	Tuesday	Wednesday	Thursday	Friday	Saturday	Sunday

THANK YOU allows you to see yourself sitting in the circles that benefit your life

Monday	Tuesday	Wednesday	Thursday	Friday	Saturday	Sunday

THANK YOU allows you to see through the lens of your mind

Monday	Tuesday	Wednesday	Thursday	Friday	Saturday	Sunday

THANK YOU allows you to view the world from a different perspective

Monday	Tuesday	Wednesday	Thursday	Friday	Saturday	Sunday

THANK YOU

Dream Realm

THANK YOU causes you to dream your wildest dream

Monday	Tuesday	Wednesday	Thursday	Friday	Saturday	Sunday

THANK YOU helps you to create from new ideas

Monday	Tuesday	Wednesday	Thursday	Friday	Saturday	Sunday

THANK YOU activates whispers from heaven to send clues for your future

Monday	Tuesday	Wednesday	Thursday	Friday	Saturday	Sunday

THANK YOU cultivate your dreams

Monday	Tuesday	Wednesday	Thursday	Friday	Saturday	Sunday

THANK YOU shapes the ideas of your dreams

Monday	Tuesday	Wednesday	Thursday	Friday	Saturday	Sunday

THANK YOU causes your dreams to proliferate and create new extensions from previous dreams

Monday	Tuesday	Wednesday	Thursday	Friday	Saturday	Sunday

THANK YOU causes your dreams to flourish

Monday	Tuesday	Wednesday	Thursday	Friday	Saturday	Sunday

THANK YOU in the physical body realm

Monday	Tuesday	Wednesday	Thursday	Friday	Saturday	Sunday

THANK YOU speaks to your cells and causes positive ions to connect to you

Monday	Tuesday	Wednesday	Thursday	Friday	Saturday	Sunday

THANK YOU allows you to use your body in a way that honors it

Monday	Tuesday	Wednesday	Thursday	Friday	Saturday	Sunday

THANK YOU allows you to reset the activities of your limbs every day for your benefit

Monday	Tuesday	Wednesday	Thursday	Friday	Saturday	Sunday

THANK YOU makes you aware of how your are feeling in your body

Monday	Tuesday	Wednesday	Thursday	Friday	Saturday	Sunday

THANK YOU makes you aware of how you're treating your body

Monday	Tuesday	Wednesday	Thursday	Friday	Saturday	Sunday

THANK YOU makes you pay attention to parts of your body that need your attention

Monday	Tuesday	Wednesday	Thursday	Friday	Saturday	Sunday

THANK YOU allows you to see your organs fully healed

Monday	Tuesday	Wednesday	Thursday	Friday	Saturday	Sunday

THANK YOU
Wealth Realm

THANK YOU causes your money to be used as seed

Monday	Tuesday	Wednesday	Thursday	Friday	Saturday	Sunday

THANK YOU activates the seed of your money to produce your ideas

Monday	Tuesday	Wednesday	Thursday	Friday	Saturday	Sunday

THANK YOU causes items to come to you versus the money

Monday	Tuesday	Wednesday	Thursday	Friday	Saturday	Sunday

Write down as many reasons to be grateful at this very present moment

_____

_____

_____

_____

_____

_____

_____

Now Say.......

THANK YOU

THANK YOU causes people to teach you how to produce the wealth

Monday	Tuesday	Wednesday	Thursday	Friday	Saturday	Sunday

THANK YOU says, "He knows our walk and He is right there with us."

Monday	Tuesday	Wednesday	Thursday all	Friday	Saturday	Sunday

THANK YOU causes people to give you their trade secrets

Monday	Tuesday	Wednesday	Thursday	Friday	Saturday	Sunday

THANK YOU causes people to pour into you

Monday	Tuesday	Wednesday	Thursday	Friday	Saturday	Sunday

THANK YOU

Peace Realm

THANK YOU activates the peace that passes all understanding.

Monday	Tuesday	Wednesday	Thursday	Friday	Saturday	Sunday

THANK YOU creates an environment of grace to have peace in the midst of your pain to understand

Monday	Tuesday	Wednesday	Thursday	Friday	Saturday	Sunday

THANK YOU stops obstacles that are blocking your peace

Monday	Tuesday	Wednesday	Thursday	Friday	Saturday	Sunday

THANK YOU creates a space for peace to be released over your circumstances

Monday	Tuesday	Wednesday	Thursday	Friday	Saturday	Sunday

THANK YOU

Respect Realm

THANK YOU signifies that you do not take them for granted.

Monday	Tuesday	Wednesday	Thursday	Friday	Saturday	Sunday

Write down as many reasons to be grateful at this very present moment

----

Now Say.......

THANK YOU

THANK YOU recognizes the Sovereignty of God's Plan for your life

Monday	Tuesday	Wednesday	Thursday	Friday	Saturday	Sunday

Now Say.......

THANK YOU

THANK YOU

Voice Realm

THANK YOU says you matter to me

Monday	Tuesday	Wednesday	Thursday	Friday	Saturday	Sunday

THANK YOU says I see the efforts you have taken to help me

Monday	Tuesday	Wednesday	Thursday	Friday	Saturday	Sunday

THANK YOU says your time and your presence mean something to my life

Monday	Tuesday	Wednesday	Thursday	Friday	Saturday	Sunday

THANK YOU says I realize you went the extra mile for me

Monday	Tuesday	Wednesday	Thursday	Friday	Saturday	Sunday

THANK YOU says I am attracting people to come to help me in my future

Monday	Tuesday	Wednesday	Thursday	Friday	Saturday	Sunday

THANK YOU says I notice you

Monday	Tuesday	Wednesday	Thursday	Friday	Saturday	Sunday

THANK YOU says I am attracting abundance to my life

Monday	Tuesday	Wednesday	Thursday	Friday	Saturday	Sunday

THANK YOU says I value you

Monday	Tuesday	Wednesday	Thursday	Friday	Saturday	Sunday

THANK YOU says I am grateful for every little thing

Monday	Tuesday	Wednesday	Thursday	Friday	Saturday	Sunday

THANK YOU says, "I am grateful for the air I breathe"

Monday	Tuesday	Wednesday	Thursday	Friday	Saturday	Sunday

THANK YOU

Work Realm

THANK YOU works to create resilience

Monday	Tuesday	Wednesday	Thursday	Friday	Saturday	Sunday

THANK YOU works to create compassion

Monday	Tuesday	Wednesday	Thursday	Friday	Saturday	Sunday

THANK YOU works to get you moving

Monday	Tuesday	Wednesday	Thursday	Friday	Saturday	Sunday

THANK YOU works to create purpose

Monday	Tuesday	Wednesday	Thursday	Friday	Saturday	Sunday

THANK YOU works to create vision

Monday	Tuesday	Wednesday	Thursday	Friday	Saturday	Sunday

THANK YOU works to create elevation

Monday	Tuesday	Wednesday	Thursday	Friday	Saturday	Sunday

THANK YOU creates the work of expansion

Monday	Tuesday	Wednesday	Thursday	Friday	Saturday	Sunday

THANK YOU creates the work of height, depth and length for your dimensional blessings

Monday	Tuesday	Wednesday	Thursday	Friday	Saturday	Sunday

116

The GIFT of a

THANK YOU

GOES A LONG WAY

Now Say.......

THANK YOU